Giselle Roeder

11/3
'12/4

Sauna

The Hottest Way to Good Health

alive books

Vancouver
Canada

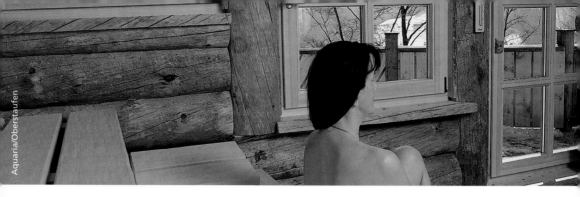

Aquaria/Oberstaufen

Contents

Note: Conversions in this book (from imperial to metric) are not exact. They have been rounded to the nearest measurement for convenience. Exact measurements are given in imperial. The recipes in this book are by no means to be taken as therapeutic. They simply promote the philosophy of both the author and *alive* books in relation to whole foods, health and nutrition, while incorporating the practical advice given by the author in the first section of the book.

Recipes

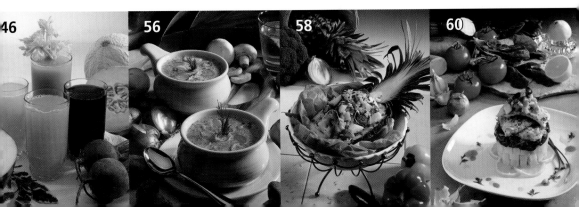
46   56   58   60

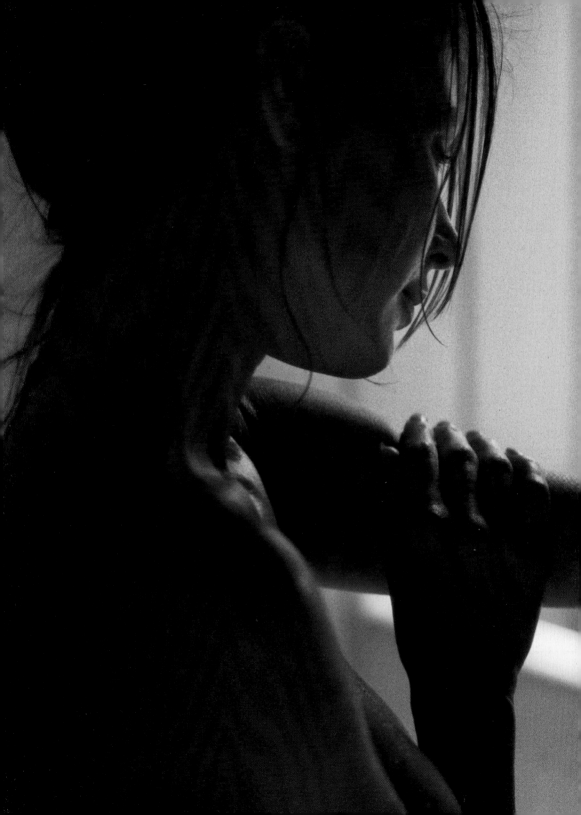

Boost immunity and prevent disease with soothing sauna sessions.

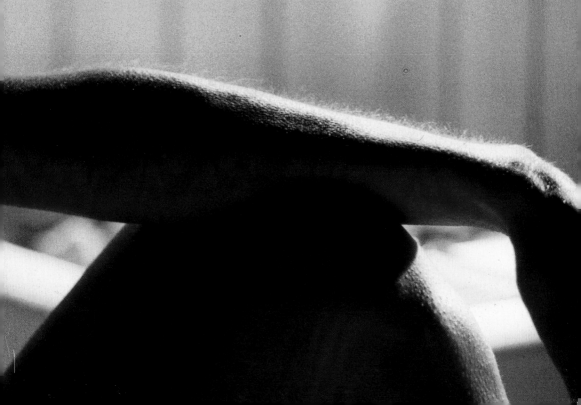

Introduction . . . .

The sauna is *not* just a place to warm up after a swim in the pool, and it's certainly not just a place to socialize with bikini-clad friends, or do business, as television commercials and movies would have us believe. What *is* the sauna? In short, it's an ancient way of cleansing the body, mind and soul. Its benefits have been enjoyed in many parts of the world for centuries. Among other benefits, people love the stress relief and the wonderful muscle relaxation that sauna brings. You too can take advantage of this ancient knowledge to feel better and relieve a variety of health problems. Whether it's a skin condition, a bad back or insomnia, or if you simply want to boost immunity to prevent disease and ailments, the sauna can help.

The sauna provides an ancient way of cleansing the body and relieving a variety of health problems.

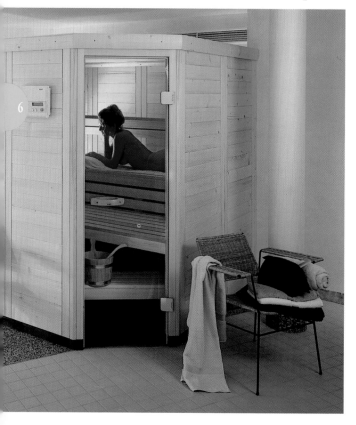

Sauna is sweating induced by high, dry heat, followed by rinsing or immersion in cold water. The process is repeated two or three times. The sauna is the only place on Earth where we can stand temperatures near 100°C (212°F). With no humidity to speak of and no restrictive clothing, the body deals with the heat by sweating profusely. This keeps the inner "core" body temperature close to the natural setting of 37°C (98.6°F). A very cold rinse or shower or a dip into a lake or a special tub stops the sweating. Originally, the "sweat bath" was a cleansing routine since warm water was not readily available.

The Wonders of Sauna

The Finns have an expression: "If spirits, tar and sauna don't help, the disease is deadly." The old proverb points to the importance of the sauna for good health. First and foremost the sauna builds up the immune system. The contrast of hot and cold "trains" the blood vessels to react quickly in order to adjust the body temperature to heat or cold. This change strengthens veins and arteries and keeps them elastic. In Finnish writings, the sauna has been referred to as a Fountain of Youth. The list of benefits derived from the sauna is seemingly endless. The following are among the many benefits:

- Provides deep, total-body cleansing
- Gives you younger-looking skin through better nourishment from within
- Speeds healing of acne and similar skin problems
- Increases and strengthens the immune system
- Reduces colds and flu
- Relieves chronic ailments of the respiratory system, such as hay fever, asthma and bronchitis
- Helps regulate high blood pressure
- Increases total circulation
- Improves heart circulation/oxygenation
- Has a protective effect on the arteries, especially important for diabetics
- Reduces muscle tension and pain
- Relieves "bad backs"
- Has a beneficial effect on rheumatism, arthritis and fibromyalgia
- Provides detoxification through better water management within the body
- Releases heavy metals from the body
- Eases pregnancy and childbirth
- Relieves stress
- Improves sleep
- Lifts depression
- Has a balancing effect on the psyche and emotions.

The sauna builds up the immune system for overall health.

7

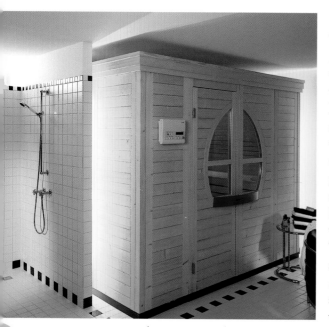

Today's sophisticated, electronically controlled saunas have come a long way since the traditional "sweat bath."

Origins of the Sauna

The Finnish sauna tradition is more than 2,000 years old, but the Finns aren't the only ones who knew the secret of sauna. It is closely related to the hot-air bath used by the Spartans, who would follow up with a dip in very cold water. Russian peasants enjoyed their *bania*, a steam bath, often taken in their baking or heating ovens, with water splashed onto hot stones. The Romans had a variety of saunas and baths, including the *balneae, thermae, tepidarium* and *laconium*. They perfected a warm-air bath in which the heat was piped in between double walls. In the 19th century, the Russian and Roman traditions were combined and became known as the Russian-Roman Bath. The Turks have their *hammam*, a steam bath with high humidity—and rigid rules.

The sweat bath, now known worldwide as the sauna, is not just an Old World custom. The Mayans and Aztecs also enjoyed sweat baths, but the Spanish invasion led to the temporary demise of this hygienic, prophylactic and healthful practice; Guatemalans and Mexicans now enjoy their *temascal.* The Japanese love their *sentoo* and *o-furo* hot-water baths. Asians and Mongols, entering what is now North America via the Bering Strait, brought their form of sweat bathing along. Some Native North Americans still use sweat lodges; it is an honor to be invited to join one.

Today, saunas run the gamut from simple sweat huts to the most sophisticated electronically controlled and multifunction facilities. But the Finnish dry hot-air sauna is considered the healthiest way to sweat. Many scientific and medical studies confirm the health benefits—but you have to do it properly!

Let's start by saying it properly: sauna is pronounced "SOWna," not "SAWna." The word "sauna," from *savne, suonje* and *suownje*, might be the only word of the Finnish language that is understood around the world. We use the Finnish name because modern knowledge of the sauna spread from Finland. It began with Finnish teams at the Olympics, and continued to spread via soldiers who learned to appreciate the sauna in Russia and Finland during World War I. Since the original Finnish sauna is a very simple hut, many of these servicemen built saunas in their home countries.

The Ultimate Sweat Bath

Extreme heat–extreme cold. That is the idea of the sauna. The sweating period takes between six and fifteen minutes; this is followed by a cool-down period of the same time. Most people do two or occasionally three sauna sessions per visit. Some people prefer the steam sauna with its high humidity because they feel they sweat more and faster. This might be an illusion since high humidity, with the air saturated with water molecules, does not allow the evaporation of sweat. The cool-down period here is very important because in the high-humidity environment the lungs and heart get overheated and have to work much harder. This is probably the reason that the much milder Roman forms of warm-air *(tepidarium)* or hot-air *(laconium)* bathing have made a come-back, especially in Italy and Austria.

Some Like It Hot: Temperatures

So, you're a reasonably healthy person and you decided to try a sauna. The first time you enter the dry Finnish sauna you might think, "I can't breathe!" It is incredibly hot. Can you imagine being comfortable in 100°C heat? And that your body can take it, that your heart won't stop beating? Believe it or not, the dry sauna, with its very low humidity of less than 10 percent on average, is in fact healthy at this high temperature. It *will* make you feel good. The biggest obstacle for the novice is the burning sensation of the hot air inhaled through the nose. Slow breathing through the mouth will ease the adjustment.

Modern saunas are usually heated electrically from the out-side. Electronic devices for temperature and humidity control, as well as for the selection of various programs, are available. A heater unit, usually located in a corner of the sauna room, is the heart of the sauna. It can sit on the floor or be mounted on the

The Finnish dry hot-air sauna is considered the healthiest way to sweat. Many scientific and medical studies confirm the health benefits.

9

wall. This unit is responsible for your comfort, the climate in the sauna, the temperature and the right heat distribution. For protection, a wooden casing or lattice fence is placed around it. Rocks are piled up around the heater element and overflow onto the top, retaining the heat very well. The top rocks also receive the occasional dousing with water to temporarily increase the humidity, and with it, the heat. Do not go into the sauna before it is ready: it takes one to two hours for the sauna to "ripen." This preparation time ensures that the wooden floor, benches, walls and ceiling absorb, retain and reflect the heat.

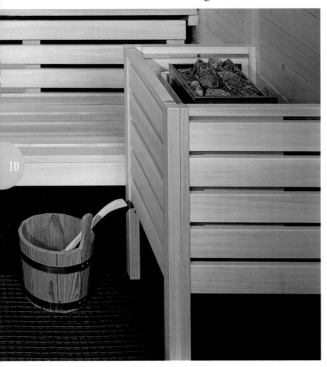

The temperature is not the same all over the sauna. Hot air expands and gets lighter, therefore it rises. The highest temperature and the lowest humidity are at the ceiling. A very low relative humidity of approximately 2 to 5 percent enables the ceiling temperature of 100°C to reflect onto your body without harm when you are on the uppermost bench (usually the third). At the surface of the third bench the temperature is about 80° to 90°C (176°–194°F); the humidity here is already a little higher than that at the ceiling– 7 to 10 percent. On the middle bench in a sauna with three benches, the temperature is about 70°C (158°F), while the humidity could be as high as 15 percent. At the lowest bench, which in a sauna with three benches is used only as a step, the temperature is about 45° to 50°C (113°–122°F)–not hot enough to induce the desired level of sweating. The humidity here is the highest, at 20 to 35 percent.

On the floor the temperature is about 40°C (104°F). The air is saturated with humidity and, through the airflow in the sauna, is forced out through a vent located in the lower part of one wall. The fresh-air ventilation system is also located in the lower area, sometimes under or behind the heater unit. The fresh air is pushed to the ceiling, absorbs the heat of the wooden walls and benches and the perspiring bodies and loses its moisture content on the way. The heavier parts of the air drift toward the bottom. The oxygen content of the air at the higher areas is lower as well. It does not, however, have the disabling effect on the body that thinner air high up on a mountain does because no muscular work or movement, which requires oxygen, is done in the sauna. In total relaxation the body uses less oxygen.

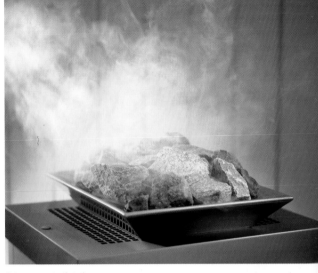

Humidity in the sauna may be temporarily increased by dousing the hot rocks with water.

Dousing the hot rocks with water temporarily increases the humidity in the whole sauna room by 10 to 15 percent. This increase feels like a blast of very hot air and can cause a burning pain. Douse the rocks to induce very heavy sweating, the body's natural reaction to heat. You can add a few drops of aromatic oil to the water to tantalize the respiratory system. Check with everyone in the sauna before dousing the rocks. Don't do this during the first sauna session; wait until the beginning of the second round, when your respiratory system and skin are totally cooled off.

How Sauna Works:
What's Happening in Your Body . . . .

The Ultimate Skin Tonic

The first contact organ in the sauna is your skin. It protects you from light and chemicals and cushions physical assaults. The first visible signs of aging are often drying and wrinkling of the skin. If you're concerned that the hot, dry sauna air will dry your skin, don't worry; it won't. Heat and water soften the top layer of skin cells, liquefy sebaceous (oily) skin secretions containing metabolic waste and attached bacteria, and sweat rinses it all away. The cooling effect of sweat evaporating on the skin releases the heat from your body. Better circulation provides moisture and nourishment for the cells, induces faster cell renewal and slows down the aging clock. The skin of a regular sauna user looks younger. The skin is also our "third kidney," taking over waste and water management if the kidneys are overloaded or not working properly.

Another important skin function is controlling the body's temperature. The body has a very accurate thermostat: the body's core temperature is kept at a steady 37°C (98.6°F). The temperature of the skin, arms and legs measures only about 32° or 33°C (90°–91°F). Your feet might be even colder. Should the body have to deal with an invasion of bacteria or a virus, the core temperature goes up by several degrees–a fever. Bugs don't like the heat and this is your body's attempt to deal with the invaders and kill them. That's why it's unwise to try to bring down a fever artificially. Except in infants, and as long as it doesn't get too high, the fever is part of our natural defense mechanism and is safe. Using the sauna does not create an artificial fever because the body's core temperature does not go up more than 1°C (less than 2°F).

Even people who claim they don't perspire will do so in the sauna, but in the very high heat and very low humidity of the sauna the initial perspiration immediately evaporates, so it might seem like you're not sweating that much at first. In as little as three minutes the body shell has

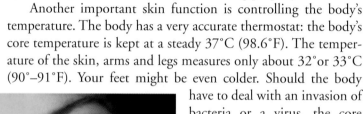

The skin of a regular sauna user looks younger due to improved circulation and cleansing.

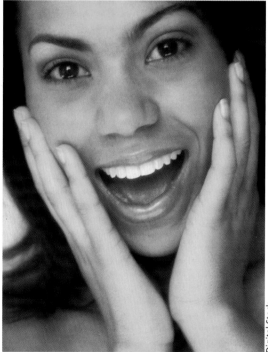

Digital Stock

heated up and the skin temperature has increased from 32° or 33°C to 40°C (104°F) and this causes more profuse sweating. You will see and feel the moisture on your skin.

Your Heart Can Take It

If you're worried about using the sauna because you have heart or circulatory problems, take the advice of Finnish cardiologists: "If you can walk to the sauna, you can use the sauna." In other words, if you cannot use your legs because of heart or circulatory problems, then the sauna is out of the question. Much medical research points to the positive effects of the sauna on the heart and circulation, if the sauna is used properly. Physiologically, the sauna puts less strain on your cardiovascular system than do many other daily activities. Through the slight heat increase within the body, the veins and arteries widen all the way into the skin. More blood is required in the pipeline and your heart's contractions become more intense to pump this extra blood out with every heartbeat. Your pulse rate might go up to approximately 120 beats per minute.

It is interesting to note that the volume of blood pumped by the heart almost doubles, but with only a 50-percent increase in beat frequency. The reason for this phenomenon is the widening of veins and arteries and the resulting loss of normal resistance. Raised blood pressure sinks. The labor of the heart becomes much easier and it works more economically. Your pulse will get faster when talking, sitting or standing in the sauna, so lie down, relax and be quiet to help your heart. Dousing the rocks with water will add another fifteen to twenty heartbeats for about one minute. A pulse rate higher than this could indicate a weakened heart muscle or other problem, and could be a contraindication for the sauna; consult your health-care provider. A general rule of thumb for the highest acceptable pulse rate is 180 (for a short time only) for healthy people and regular sauna users and 180 minus your age for seniors.

Different people have different normal heart rates. The smaller the heart, the higher the pulse: at rest, a baby has a normal pulse of 120 to 130, a child 100 to 120 and an adult 60 to 80. Marathon runners or other high-performance athletes can have counts between 40 and 60. In the sauna, you will have an increase of approximately 50 percent. If you want to make sure your pulse is not too high in the sauna, you should know your average resting pulse before using the sauna.

Coronary Problems

A ten-year study in Finland, encompassing 40,000 sauna visits by people after heart attacks, noted not a single heart problem caused by the sauna. Heat and muscle relaxation affects the coronary system as well. The widening of the arteries surrounding the heart eases the pumping work and the blood flow, providing better oxygenation in the process. Having had a heart attack is not a reason to avoid the sauna, as long as you use it correctly and your health-care provider approves. Naturally, the sauna should not be used right away after a heart attack, and moderation is sensible.

High Blood Pressure

The higher the pulse, the lower the blood pressure.
The positive effect of the sauna on lowering blood pressure has led to its inclusion in the rehabilitation process for some hypertension patients. Both the systolic pressure (the first number in a blood pressure reading) during the draining of the heart chambers and the diastolic pressure (the second number) during the refilling of the heart chambers will decrease through the total relaxation of the circulation throughout the body, especially in the respiratory system and the skin. This decrease will remain during the cool-down phase even if full immersion in cold water is avoided. The normal reaction of the blood vessels to cold water is a strong contraction. The use of cold water after the hot sauna is paramount.

People with high blood pressure should use a hose, such as the one used for Kneipp water therapy, to direct the cold water from the feet up toward the heart. A cold shower from above onto the back or chest is too much of a shock and often constricts the breathing. Full immersion in a tub of cold water adds hydrostatic pressure from the outside and brings the blood pressure up. Avoid the cold immersion tub if you have hypertension. Regular sauna visits contribute to stabilization of high blood pressure if the sauna is done right. For more information on Kneipp water therapy, read *Healing with Water: Kneipp Hydrotherapy at Home*, (*alive* Natural Health Guide #11, 2000).

Low Blood Pressure

Low blood pressure responds to the sauna in a different way. During the sauna the pressure normalizes despite the relaxation within the system and the widening of the vessels. Medical research indicates that there is a release into the system of blood that was previously stored and not moving around. A person with low blood pressure has to be very careful when sitting up to get ready to leave the sauna room. It is very important to sit up slowly, put the feet on the lower bench and do "muscle pumping" (by pressing one foot after the other onto the next lower bench as if you were walking) to avoid a sudden rush of blood into the widened vessels of the legs. Dizziness and fainting spells are much more common in people with low blood pressure. After a few minutes, cool down in fresh air; immersion in a tub of cool water is allowed. To tone your circulatory system if you have hypotension, use Kneipp hydrotherapy on a daily basis. The sauna alone is not enough to alleviate low-pressure problems.

A person with low blood pressure can benefit from the sauna, but must be careful to move slowly when leaving the sauna.

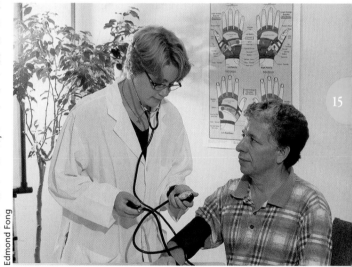

Edmond Fong

The Respiratory System

Your respiratory system, right from the nose to the lungs, handles the heat quite well by altering the temperature of the inhaled air. It warms it up in winter and tries to cool it down in the sauna's heat. As long as the humidity is low when you enter the sauna room (long before or long after the dousing of the rocks), the dry heat presents no problem. Moist, humid heat does! I find it easier to adjust to the hot air by slowly "slurping" it through my mouth until I lie down and then carefully start breathing through my nose. Tiny blood vessels abound in the breathing pathway. Their circulation increases up to seven times and the mucous membranes add moisture to the inhaled air to cool it to match the inner body temperature. The heat is absorbed and transported into the cooler parts of the body. The production of nasal mucus increases and so does your production of immune globulin A. Scientists believe that this, combined with the contrast of hot and cold, means that regular sauna users have fewer respiratory-tract infections.

Asthma and chronic bronchitis sufferers find relief in the sauna. The overall relaxation of the muscular system opens up the breathing channels. Asthma attacks have not been observed in the sauna, but delay using the sauna after an attack for several days or even weeks, depending on the severity of the attack. One aspect of sauna use is particularly important for those with respiratory problems: Since the air in the sauna contains less oxygen, the inhalation of fresh air right after the sauna and before the cold-water treatments is very important. Oxygen has to be replenished and the mucous membranes need reinforcement through cooling.

The sauna experience will give you the wonderful feeling that all is right with the world.

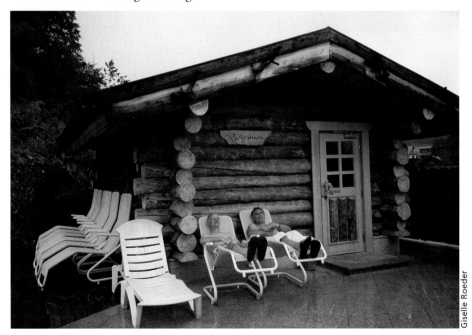

Giselle Roeder

Detoxification

Your blood contains 56 percent liquids and 44 percent cells. The blood gets thicker when part of the fluid is removed through sweating. One hour after the complete sauna session the balance is regained, even if you don't top up your fluids by drinking. It is important to note that to maintain this balance within the blood, more intercellular liquid is transferred to the blood. This also means that toxins present in the intercellular liquid are transferred into the blood stream and will then be delivered to the excretion organs–the liver and kidneys. If you drink during the sauna sessions, the liquid passes through the stomach and intestinal tract very quickly and is picked up by the blood. This undermines the detoxification process since extra intercellular fluid is then not needed by the blood.

Toxins, especially heavy metals such as copper, cadmium, lead and zinc, are picked up during the transfer and redistribution of body fluids. The blood transports these to your body surface and releases them into the thousands of tiny vessels surrounding the sweat glands. The sweat glands pick up the heavy metals and dispose of them through sweat and evaporation. Japanese studies in industrial centers confirm the detoxification of heavy metals through sweating in the sauna.

You might be wondering if you lose minerals in the sauna along with fluids and toxins. You do, but the loss is minimal: 98 to 99 percent of sauna-generated sweat is pure water, unlike the sweat produced through muscular work or sports. Half of the 1 or 2 percent that is minerals is salt; the other half is made up of other minerals plus lactic acid, lipid acid, uric acid and heavy metal toxins. This mineral loss is easily replaced after the sauna with fruit juice, a fresh salad or mineral water.

Stress Management

"Anger goes up in smoke and the gall bladder dries out in the sauna." This Finnish proverb points to another benefit of the sauna: you can't stay mad in the sauna. Mental ease follows physical relaxation. If you do it right, the sauna experience will give you the wonderful feeling that all is right with the world. The time you spend in the sauna, the time you spend in the fresh air and the time you spend doing cold-water treatments all depend

Japanese studies in industrial centers confirm the detoxification of heavy metals through sweating in the sauna.

on how you feel. When you feel you've had enough heat, leave the sauna. When you feel you have replenished the missing oxygen, begin the water treatments, using water as cold as you feel is right for you. Do the total immersion or just use the hose or shower. What feels right is right for you.

However, you must follow the basic rule about the cold after the heat. Your good feelings will be the indicator of how much the sauna can do for you. The changes between hot and cold are stimulating to both your nervous systems–the autonomic or parasympathetic (unconscious, self-regulating) and the somatic or sympathetic (conscious, responsible for voluntary movement). The parasympathetic nervous system begins to adjust as soon as you are in the sauna. The widening of the blood vessels, lessening of muscle tension and the sweating mechanism are activated. Once the core temperature starts to rise a little, the sympathetic nervous system adds a feeling of restlessness, including a faster pulse. You will soon feel it is time to get out. The cold-water treatments employ both nervous systems again to reverse the process: blood vessels tighten up and the heartbeat normalizes. The parasympathetic system temporarily retreats and the sympathetic system remains in effect. An incredible feeling of refreshment and relaxation is the result.

The hot part of the sauna is often over-rated and the cold part under-rated, but the heat would not have the desired effect on the body without the cold treatments. Warm water and heat are good relaxants, but used by themselves, or with water that is not cold enough, the changes they cause can lead to damage in the affected

The sauna is soothing for the stressed mind. The hot and cold ritual is stimulating to the nervous system, easing both the conscious and unconscious.

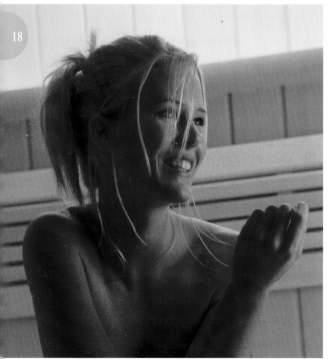

organs and to early aging. When sauna is done right, however, there is an interplay between the two parts of the nervous system. Through the influence of the parasympathetic system the pulse and heartbeat frequency remain slow for hours after the sauna. This is why you shouldn't do physical activity (working out, using fitness equipment or swimming) during the rest period.

Who Can Benefit from the Sauna? . . . .

Pregnant Women

Pregnancy is not a reason for the regular sauna user to stop visiting. Finnish, German and American studies confirm this. "Birthing is easy for the new mother if the sauna is heated up with the wood of trees hit by lightning." So say the folk tales of Finland. In old times, when the sauna was heated with wood (the smoke sauna) it provided some degree of protection against infection. Since saunas in those days had no chimneys, the benches, floor and walls got covered with soot during heating. The sauna then had to be scrubbed before use and was therefore one of the cleanest places around.

The greatest benefit of the sauna for pregnant women is better water management within the body. During pregnancy, approximately eight liters (eight quarts) of extra water is maintained in your body and your blood volume increases by more than 30 percent. Many women feel their shoes or rings getting too tight during pregnancy. The sauna helps to decrease swelling caused by water retention since excess water is released through sweating. Pregnant women have to deal with their own metabolic waste as well as those of their babies; sweating helps remove more toxins that would otherwise be stored in the tissues.

Another sauna benefit for pregnant women is the training of blood vessels through the contrast of hot and cold. Varicose veins, often caused by pregnancy, are prevented. Blood flow, which is slower during pregnancy, increases. This provides better oxygenation throughout the body. In certain cases, worry about thrombosis is reduced. Cramping is reduced. Great psychological benefits are achieved through the total relaxation brought on by the sauna; it is a good way to prepare for labor. Many women who use the sauna find that their labors are shorter and stress is reduced.

Users pregnant for the first time are advised to wait until after the fifteenth week of pregnancy before using the sauna. Only if you are carrying more than one baby or if you have serious health concerns should you avoid using the sauna during your pregnancy. Women with a tendency to give birth before term should not use the sauna during the last three months of their pregnancies. And needless to say, all pregnant women should use the sauna with discretion with regard to temperature and time. You should continue to use the cold-water cool down, just avoid the cold-water immersion tub.

Men and Fertility

Men who have concerns about their fertility can benefit from the sauna. Statistics prove that it is the male partner who is infertile in approximately one third of couples who cannot conceive. Medical studies confirm that the sperm-producing organs are very temperature sensitive. The testicles are located outside of the body so that their temperature can be maintained at about 2°C (less than 4°F) lower than the body's core temperature. Frequent hot bathing and long stays in hot whirlpools reduce the production and motility of sperm. However, studies prove that the dry sauna heat does not have the same effect. On the contrary, the proper use of the sauna increases the concentration of testosterone in the blood; fertility can increase along with it. However, note that wearing a bathing suit in the sauna traps too much heat around the body and is counterproductive.

Studies show that while the hot tub decreases fertility, the dry heat of the sauna increases the concentration of testosterone in the blood and fertility along with it.

Children

Children naturally love the sauna and everything to do with water. Children over the age of two years can handle the heat quite well because of the elasticity in their circulatory systems. The increase in body temperature is negligible. Children have the same number of sweat glands as adults do and their bodies deal with the

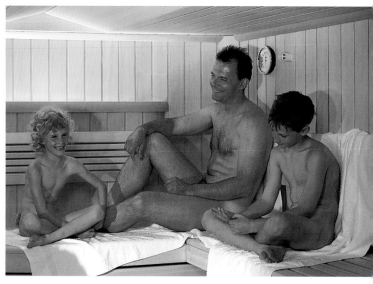

heat easily. Studies with kindergarten-age children showed an increase in immune function, fewer colds and a greater awareness of hygiene in children who use the sauna.

Children should lie on the second bench rather than on the top bench. The time in the sauna is the same as for adults and allows the parents to observe their children. Watch that children do not overdo the cold-water treatments and become chilled since they do not seem to feel the cold water the way adults do.

Children have the same number of sweat glands that adults do. Those more than two years of age can deal with the heat of the sauna easily.

Seniors

Unless you have serious health concerns, there is no age limit for the sauna. A slower metabolism and functional changes in circulation and hormone production, and especially the loss of intercellular fluids, cause the signs of aging. The sauna can be part of a rejuvenation program.

People who start using the sauna before they reach their senior years are at an advantage, but it's never too late to start. Do, however, check with your health-care provider first if you are older and have any health concerns. Heavy sweating helps remove waste contained in the cells and improves mobility. The skin gets a thorough moisturizing from within and cells are "bathed." The increase in skin temperature by 10°C (17°F) and better circulation fosters cell renewal. Regular sauna visits, with their hot-cold contrast, train the blood vessels and prevent circulation problems. Since the sauna's heat does not influence your skin's oil glands, older people, who tend to have drier skin, should apply skin lotion after the sauna. And drink lots of fluids!

What Sauna Is *Not* . . . .

Champagne, Socializing and Weight Loss

Before I describe in detail the steps of the sauna ritual, I'd like to dispel some of the myths that surround the sauna. Lots of people look forward to meeting their friends and socializing with them during sauna sessions. Those who have a home sauna might invite their friends to enjoy a sauna with them. They might even have a few drinks before stepping into the sauna; sometimes glasses of champagne are taken into the sauna room. But drinking alcohol before or during a sauna is not good for your health! It affects your brain, circulation and blood pressure, as well as the detoxification efforts of the liver and kidneys and the removal of heavy metals via perspiration. Alcohol in any form is bad news for sauna users–don't drink and sweat!

Socializing in the sauna–without alcohol–might be all right for a family who uses their sauna every night to relax or talk about the day's events. However, if the sauna is used for health purposes, try to refrain from talking. The Finns regard the sauna as an almost sacred place. You must behave accordingly: no shouting, quarreling or loud conversation. Aside from disturbing others, conversation alters your mindset, changes your blood pressure and prevents normal relaxation. You cannot achieve the full benefit of the sauna while you're chatting. Save the talking until you're finished. Then, you'll feel refreshed and ready to socialize.

When we think of socializing at the sauna, we might also think of hot tubs or whirlpools, often known as Jacuzzis®. But hot tubs and saunas definitely don't mix. Never use them during the same session unless just for a five minute warm footbath. In fact, use hot tubs with caution even if you're not having a sauna–they can be dangerous if you spend too much time in them. Because you are almost entirely submerged in hot water, when your body heats up it can't disperse the heat. In extreme cases, you could be in danger of a stroke. If you do use a hot tub, don't spend more than fifteen minutes in it, and remember that cold-water treatments to cool down afterward are essential. And as in the sauna, avoid alcohol!

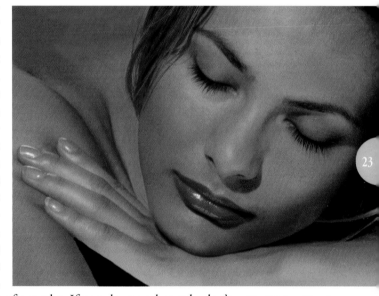

The full benefits of a healthful sauna cannot be achieved if you are talking. Quiet relaxation is best.

Sweating It Off: Another Sauna Myth

Weight loss is *not* one of the benefits of the sauna. The increase in the activity of the metabolism is not great enough to cause weight reduction. You can weigh yourself before you start the sauna and again afterward, and you might notice the loss of up to two pounds, but this is due to heavy sweating. Your body's fluids have been used to keep cool.

Although you might be one to two pounds lighter after your sauna, you haven't lost any fat, just water. After the sauna you will be thirsty. The lost liquid has to be replaced to avoid serious health consequences. Trying to "sweat off the weight," as is sometimes done by weight-dependent athletes, will weaken you and damage your organs.

Remember, the sauna can't help you if you don't use it correctly. Avoid the following in relation to your sauna:

- A hectic and stressful schedule and hurrying through sauna sessions
- Going into the sauna with a wet body or bathing suit
- Skipping the cold water necessary to cool down between sauna sessions
- Drinking or eating during sauna sessions
- Sitting upright in the sauna with legs hanging down
- Exercising (swimming, working out) between or after sauna sessions
- Returning to the sauna without being outside long enough to cool down
- Failing to allow enough fresh air between sauna sessions to replace oxygen
- Using a hot tub between or after sauna sessions
- Talking, reading or exercising in the sauna.

How To Take a Sauna . . . .

Now that you know why you need to use the sauna, let's look at the proper way to do it. There's more to it than simply sweating!

Birthday Suit or Bikini?

Nudity in the sauna is considered totally natural and has never been associated with sexuality.

In Europe, nudity in the sauna is considered totally natural and has never been associated with sexuality. Among family and close friends of whatever age, shape or sex, the lack of clothing in the sauna is not an issue at all. In public saunas, however, men and women often have different bathing days, though in central Europe mixed sauna days are very common.

Why is nudity important? The body regulates the heat assault on the skin and keeps the core temperature steady. The

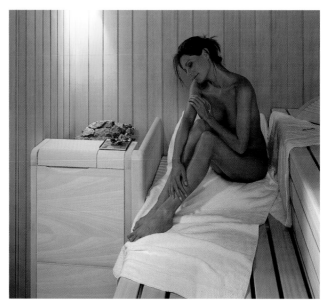

"SOS" sent to the brain by the skin is answered by widening the arteries and sending more blood to the legs, arms and skin; this causes perspiration within two to three minutes. In the dry heat and low humidity of the Finnish sauna, this first perspiration evaporates immediately. To provide the cooling effect necessary the body starts serious sweating. You lose about 10 grams of water per minute. Within the sixty to ninety minutes of a two- or three-session sauna bath you can lose up to one liter (one quart) of water.

If you wear a bathing suit in the sauna it will trap heat next to your skin; evaporation cannot take place and your skin will heat to an uncomfortable temperature.

A bathing suit will trap heat next to your skin. Evaporation cannot take place underneath clothing and your skin will heat up too much. I once had to leave a sauna because my bikini top became so hot that I couldn't stand it. Most of our two million sweat glands are located on the torso, with fewer on the arms and legs. In the worst-case scenario, a full bathing suit made of artificial fiber covering most of the torso could cause a stroke since your body does not have adequate release for the heat. The respiratory pathways get hot, the inhaled air is hot, your core temperature is already up and if the body overheats by even half a degree it could be very dangerous.

So if because of culture or custom it is not possible to wear your birthday suit, wear the smallest bikini or bathing trunks, made of light unlined cotton, that you can find. If you have to shower and cool down in it as well, have two outfits. Do not keep the wet one on to re-enter the sauna. Change into a dry garment to help your body with its temperature control and to keep sweating. Never go into the sauna with a wet body or wet swimsuit. You will not sweat until the moisture on your skin has evaporated.

What You Need for a Sauna

Pack a bag with the following items:

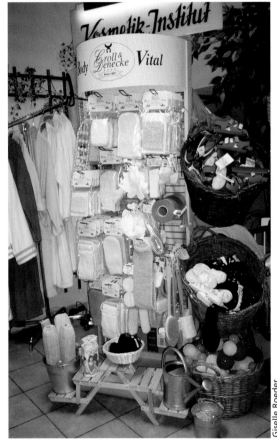

Giselle Roeder

Be prepared for your sauna session by packing a bag with necessities.

Two or three towels: You need a towel to dry yourself after the initial cleansing shower. While in the sauna you need one towel that is long enough to lie down on, head to toe. The third towel comes in handy after the cold-water immersions, rinses, showers and foot baths in between sauna sessions.

A bathrobe: Use this for the recommended resting time after the cleansing shower before you enter the sauna and after the cooling-off period. Avoid becoming chilled.

Slippers: Find a pair with wooden or soft rubber soles. These will prevent you from picking up any fungus at a public sauna and from getting chilled on the tiled floor outside the sauna. Wear your slippers into the sauna, then leave them on the sauna floor when you step up onto the benches. Put them back on when you leave the sauna to go to the cooling-off area. In a public sauna you might want to keep your slippers on during the shower and other water treatments.

Soap, shampoo, hairdryer, body lotion and dry-brush: Use soap and shampoo during the cleansing shower prior to your sauna. If your hair is thick and full or too long to towel-dry, use a hairdryer after drying your body. You may dry-brush your body before you enter the sauna. This speeds up the perspiration process and helps to cleanse and regenerate the skin.

Clean clothing: The sauna is a deep-cleansing bath. Put on fresh, clean clothing when you are finished.

23 Steps to the Perfect Sauna . . . .

Here, then, are the steps to successful, rejuvenating, healthful sauna:

1. Have a light meal before you visit the sauna. Light soup, salad or some fruit will do. If you are hungry in the sauna you might feel weak and sick; an overloaded stomach does not allow for detoxification since too much blood is needed for digestion. It is important not to eat or drink anything once you have started the sauna process. Sweating activates detoxification in your body. Many toxins, including heavy metals, are eliminated through the skin. Eating or drinking will disrupt the process.

2. Empty your bowels less than twenty-four hours prior to your sauna; void your bladder just prior to using the sauna.

3. Remove all jewelry. Metal heats up quickly and will burn you.

4. Shower with warm water, soap and shampoo. Dry your body and hair completely.

5. Dry-brush your whole body from the feet up to the neck to promote faster sweating.

6. Rest, covered with your bathrobe, until your pulse is normal.

7. Take a warm foot bath (ankle deep) for five minutes; dry your feet.

8. Enter the sauna slowly; close the door behind you. Stand for a moment to adjust your breathing, then remove your slippers.

9. Step slowly onto the first bench.

10. Lie down, on your towel, on the second or third bench. Your head should be slightly elevated on one of the wooden headrests. If there is not enough room to stretch out, pull your feet toward you or lie on your side with your feet on

Do not sit with your feet hanging down. Your whole body must be at the same level.

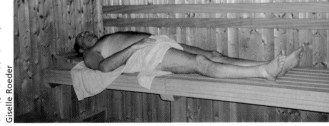

Giselle Roeder

27

the same bench. *Do not* sit with your feet hanging down. Your whole body must be at the same level. When you sit up your head is in a hotter zone than your bottom is. You could become light-headed as a result.

11. Look at the clock, relax, close your eyes. Give yourself over to the warmth penetrating your body. Do not move. Do not talk. Breathe evenly. You will not notice your perspiration for the first few minutes since it immediately evaporates. Certain areas, such as your face, knees and shins, might feel too hot because they have few sweat glands. Use your hands to transfer some perspiration from other areas. This first session should not be longer than eight to twelve minutes.

12. Get up slowly after about twelve minutes, or at the slightest feeling of unease or dizziness. Lower your feet to the bench below and sit for two to three minutes to adjust the circulation. Do some "foot pumping": press both feet onto the lower bench. Alternating feet, raise one heel while keeping the ball of the foot firmly on the bench. The muscle action will help to tighten up the blood vessels so that the blood will be pumped back into the body from the legs. Too much blood in the widened vessels of the legs and not enough in the brain can cause dizziness and sometimes even fainting. You need to adjust to the vertical position before you get up. Breathe evenly and then slowly climb down, take your towel with you, put on your slippers and leave the sauna room. Don't hurry.

A breath of fresh air after a sauna is valuable for cooling down the respiratory system and replenishing oxygen.

28

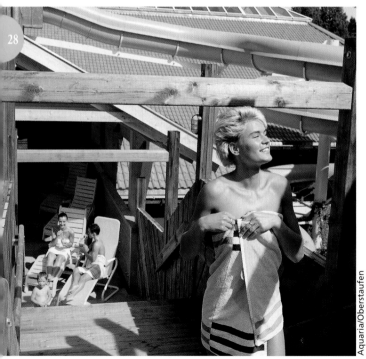

Aquaria/Oberstaufen

13. Breathe some fresh air, move around and walk a bit, outside if possible, for several minutes. This is important for cooling down the respiratory system and replenishing oxygen, which is reduced in the sauna. Expose your body to the air. If necessary, hold your towel around you loosely. The veins in your legs are still wider and too much blood can sink into them again if you stand still. A shortage of blood and oxygen in your head and upper body could result. By walking, the muscles will keep the blood moving. If you cannot go outside but can breathe some fresh air through an open window, do so, but keep walking "on the spot."

The heat of the sauna would not have the desired effect on the body without the cold treatments that follow.

14. Apply cold water from the feet up. Use a hose with a wide opening if available. The water should be really cold and cover the skin like a mantle; there should be no air trapped in the water. Start at the farthest spot from the heart–your right baby toe. Move up the leg to the hip on the outside and back down on the inside of the leg; repeat on your left leg. Now point the water into your right hand, move it up to the shoulder and let it run over the right half of your body, moving the hose back and forth covering front and back. Move down on the inside of the right arm. Do the same with the left arm. Now bend forward, point the water at your chest and make a figure eight several times. Straighten up and run the water up the right leg again. Make a spiral around the abdomen starting on the lower right side. Rinse your face; make sure to run the water behind your ears as well. The Finns recommend that the cold water run over your head as well.

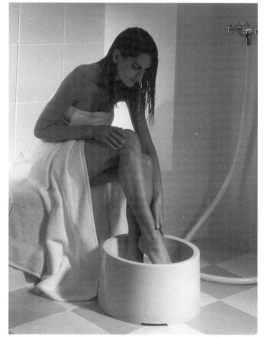

Use the shower if there is no hose available. Step slowly into the cold water. Let it first cover your feet, legs and hips, then your whole body.

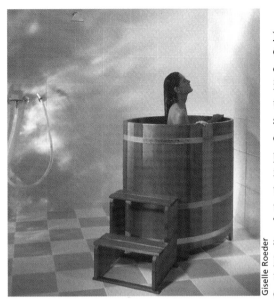

After using the shower or hose you can immerse yourself in a tub of cold water to provide a total cool down. However, only strong, healthy individuals or experienced sauna users should do this. Note that you should not do this full immersion in cold water if you have high blood pressure because during this treatment your body deals not only with the cold temperature but also with the hydrostatic pressure of the water. This brings the blood pressure up and will have a negative impact on people already dealing with hypertension. If in doubt, ask your health-care provider.

Giselle Roeder

Strong, healthy, experienced sauna users can derive great benefits from total immersion in a tub of cold water after a sauna.

Take about twelve to fifteen minutes to cool down. This can include a resting period lying down covered with a towel or bathrobe. *Do not* exercise or swim immediately after the sauna session.

15. **Have another warm foot bath** for five minutes. Dry your feet.

16. **Go back into the sauna** as before. Use the third (top) bench this time if you used the second bench before. Repeat steps 10 to 15.

17. **Repeat a third time** if you are an experienced sauna user.

18. **Cool down completely** after the last sauna session; make sure that no more sweating occurs and your body is at ease, the pulse normal and a general feeling of great health has taken hold of you. Walk around and breathe fresh air to replenish oxygen while you gently exercise the blood vessels in your legs. Do the cold rinse or cold tub immersion and completely dry your body. Slip into your robe and have another warm foot bath, dry your feet and rub lotion into your skin, especially into your legs and the soles of your feet. Wear long socks to keep your feet warm. It is important for your body to retain its normal temperature and not get chilled. That can happen easily if you lie down, for

example in a meditation room or outside in a lawn chair. I once went to a "dreamland meditation room" featuring a changing night sky with only my sauna towel, and got chilled. Also, note that your skin is now very sensitive, deeply clean and much more prone to sunburn.

19. Replenish lost fluids. After the last cool down and before resting and/or massage, have a tall glass of mineral or spring water, fruit juice or vegetable juice. Fresh-pressed carrot or mixed vegetable juice with a teaspoon of flaxseed or olive oil is ideal. Avoid very cold drinks because your digestive tract is still heated. And no alcohol! Your body has detoxified and through sweating used a lot of intercellular fluids. The blood is thicker and needs to normalize. Fluids taken from organs and other tissues have to be replaced. (If you are on lithium therapy it is very important to drink right after finishing the sauna, even before the cool-down period.)

Edmond Fong

Fluids lost through detoxification in the sauna can be replaced by drinking healthful juices or mineral water following your final cool down.

When you drink, do not gulp the liquid. Keep it in your mouth for a few seconds, roll it around and then swallow it sip by sip. Your stomach will appreciate this warm-up, as well as the addition of enzymes from your saliva, and not go into "knots" or give you pain. The first glass of liquid will very quickly pass into the system. Have a second glass during the resting period.

20. A massage is beneficial after the final cool down and rest. After the sauna, your muscles are soft and couldn't be better prepared for massage. The massage room should be warm and the therapist should cover the parts of your body not being worked on.

21. Rest and meditate for half to three quarters of an hour in a meditation room if available, or outdoors, wearing your bathrobe;

cover your feet with your towel. Lying in a lounge chair in a garden, in winter or summer, and breathing fresh air is preferable as long as your body remains naturally warm and comfortable. Resist the temptation to read as it changes the blood distribution.

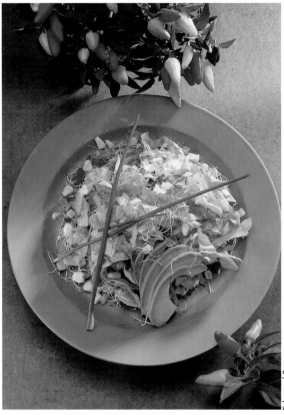

22. Get dressed in clean clothes when your body temperature has normalized and you are no longer sweating.

23. Have a light meal. After the approximately three quarters to one hour of resting, massage and meditation, you may eat something like a salad, vegetable soup or small pasta dish. You can have a slightly salty snack, but avoid sweets, cakes, cookies and chocolate. Later in the evening, if you have dinner and you feel like it, you may have beer but no wine. Do not overeat on your sauna day.

Edmond Fong

A light meal or snack, about one hour after the sauna session, is refreshening.

It's a Time Investment

Ideally, a healthful, enjoyable sauna session takes two to three hours. Do not be in a hurry when you go to the sauna. Cut out the stress, let your body calm down and normalize your heartbeat, especially if you came by bike, exercised or plan to swim before your sauna. If you want to use fitness equipment prior to your sauna, plan some extra time. Do all physical activity before and not during or after the sauna. The sauna helps to prevent or alleviate sore muscles, so it is very much appreciated by athletes.

The sauna's effects on your body last about seven days, so set aside the same time every week for your sauna. Once you are used to the sauna, you can go twice a week. If you have to rush through the sessions, then it is better not to go at all. The time spent will bring dividends only by following the rituals and not rushing. If you feel tired and worn out after the sauna you did something wrong!

Saunas Galore: The Choice Is Yours . . . .

It was not all that long ago that modern hygiene luxuries, such as hot and cold running water available at a touch, were mere dreams. When I was a child, very few families had bathrooms with bathtubs.

In European cities after the World War II, "city baths" were installed. These buildings had a number of change rooms and bathtubs. For a price one could have a nice, warm, clean private bath in a big bathtub for forty-five minutes. In time, saunas were added.

Finland, with its 5.1 million inhabitants, has more than 1.6 million saunas; the sauna has been part of Finnish life for 2,000 years. Most families have their own saunas. Many apartment buildings, and even individual apartments, have saunas. Public and club saunas are very common; all hotels have saunas. Cruise ships and freighters have them, too. Even the Finnish Legislature building has a sauna!

The International Sauna Association and the Finnish Sauna Association have very strict definitions for what a sauna is and condemn "all sorts of artificial devices which have nothing to do with the sauna but are marketed under the name. These paraphernalia vary from plastic sweating pants to a tent bag which is slipped to the neck and can be worn in the living room while watching TV" (Pirkko Valtakari, *Finnish Sauna Culture*).

That being said, there are a variety of legitimate sauna types. Try several to find the one that's right for you. Sauna is a very personal experience and you need to find out what makes you feel good. That's the secret of the sauna: it has to make you feel good. That applies to the whole experience–temperature, time, type, cool down–everything.

Public Saunas

Public saunas have become widespread all over the world as people have come to appreciate the health benefits of sweat bathing. There are incredible bath and swim complexes in Europe with everything you could dream of: swimming pools, hot tubs, water slides, wave action and whirlpools, wild water tunnels, and of course, every kind of sauna, even one with a 360-degree alpine panorama and meditative music, the sound of waterfalls in the background and color therapy. You can tan on an "electric beach," in the fresh air or meditate under a starry sky in the middle of the day. A dreamland hardly imaginable!

One such place is Aquaria in Oberstaufen, Germany. A number of the photographs in this book were taken there. What impressed me most was the "Saunascape." I could choose the traditional Finnish sauna, try several variations of it or sweat it out in the steam bath. There were separate saunas for men and women and for mixed use. Naturally there was a row of showers, stations with the Kneipp hose for cold-water body rinses, several types of immersion tubs and a long row of seats for the warm foot bath. It was also possible to go outside to cool down.

An important element usually found in public saunas in Europe is a type of shower with a wide "smiling" mouth gushing cold water. The even flow of the gushing water surrounds the body with a water "mantle" with no air trapped in it like in an ordinary shower. This is similar to a rinse with the Kneipp hose, but much more powerful. It reminded me of the almost hypnotic flow of water at Niagara Falls.

Private Saunas

Private saunas are a great way to enjoy the many benefits of the sweat bath. They can be built in all kinds of spaces: in the basement, in the attic, beside a bathroom, in the garage. If you have a garden, you can build a separate sauna hut. It could even be built into a simple tool shed. Ready-to-assemble sauna kits are available. Build your sauna outdoors, and you have easy access to the fresh air for the all-important replenishment of oxygen, winter and summer. Plant high shrubs around it for privacy and you're ready to go. Depending on where you live, you could even experience rolling in the snow after the sauna. I promise, the snow

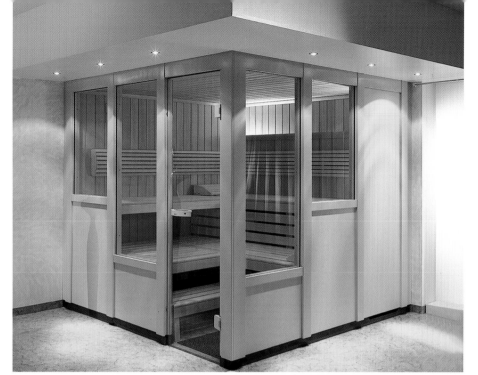

does not feel cold! As long as your body is hot it feels great. As long as the cold treatments are of short duration, you won't get chilled.

Private saunas are a wonderful way to derive the benefits of sweating.

Get all the advice you can before you decide to build a sauna yourself. The placement of the door is important. It needs to open outward so that if anyone feels dizzy and needs to leave quickly, it is possible to "fall" out of the sauna room if necessary. Check the placement of the air vents (intake and exhaust) and make sure you have a good seal all around. Don't scrimp on the heater or the control unit.

Don't forget that the sauna is an alternate form of bathing and that the change between hot and cold is important. Plan for cold-water facilities as well as a cool-down and resting room next to your sauna. A regular shower, the "gushing" shower or a hose with a wide opening, as well as a foot bath container, are essential.

I have talked to several sauna builders and the general consensus is that it is better to have the sauna built by an experienced professional to avoid costly mistakes. If not built correctly, heat and humidity could cause a problem, especially if the sauna is located in the house. I would recommend one of the pre-cut sauna kits. For use in my own house I would definitely choose the

Good Wood

If you are building your own sauna, choosing the right wood is critical. In Finland, mostly pine is used. It is good for the walls and the ceiling but has to be carefully selected for the benches because it contains many knots and these are very dense and get very hot. Sit on one and you could burn a tattoo into your derrière! Redwood or red cedar, which is less dense than pine, is often used in California. Red cedar contains cedrene, a volatile oil belonging to the terpine family, and cedral, a cedar camphor, which give it durability to withstand humidity, insect infestations and rot. But it has its drawbacks: its volatility, and its scent, which can be highly irritable and toxic to some people and can cause allergies. Aspen is a good choice since it is less dense and has fewer knots and nice straight lines. Scandinavian pine and Canadian hemlock are virtually resin-free, are durable and are conducive to a pleasant climate in the sauna. The choice of wood is also a matter of aesthetics. The growth rings in pine are not as regular as those in hemlock and therefore have a much livelier look.

For the benches and the headrests select knot-free softwood because these woods conduct negligible amounts of heat, are resin-free and contain no sap. All timber used in the sauna has to be air seasoned and chamber dried to prevent cracks and render it perfect for sauna building.

Finnish-type sauna since it provides low humidity and dry heat. Mold, fungus and rot would not be a danger to the house—or its inhabitants.

Another option is the Klafs Sauna control unit, with which you can turn the sauna into every type of sweat bath. Heat and humidity are controlled automatically. You need good ventilation for this unit.

The Dry or Finnish Sauna

Developed over the course of 2,000 years, the Finnish sauna graduated from a hole or pit dug into a slope or the ground into the wood-paneled room with benches with which we are familiar today. Originally, rocks were heated in a fire pit. Water sprinkled on the rocks raised the heat and allowed for sweating, which cleaned the body. The use of rocks and the custom of sprinkling water on them survived and is still practiced today. Writings from the 12th century mention that saunas were separate from dwellings because of the danger of fire. Thankfully, this is no longer a problem!

During the Middle Ages a new, more advanced, ground sauna was developed, featuring a roof supported by beams and a front wall of logs with a door. This type of sauna is so effective that it is still being built today. But the Finns loved their *savusauna*, the smoke sauna, best. The rocks on the stove of the *savusauna* were heated with wood and the resulting smoke blackened the room with soot before it found its way out through a vent or the slightly open door. The smoke left a distinct aroma. Charcoal formed by the soot resisted bacteria; that, combined with the fact that the floor and seating area were washed before bathing, made the sauna the most hygienic room around. The *savusauna* took a long time to heat, often burned down and the cleaning took a lot of time, but sauna connoisseurs still consider the smoke sauna superior to all other types. The Finnish Sauna Association maintains one for its members and guests. If you travel to Finland stop in Helsinki and check it out!

Cottage saunas built near the sea, a lake or river are plentiful. After the sweat bath the bather jumps into the water to cool down, summer or winter. Rolling in the snow and walking about in below-freezing temperatures without clothing after the heating doesn't make you cold, nor does it cause you to catch a cold. When the procedure is done right the immune system is actually enhanced.

The Finnish saunas with which we are most familiar are wood-paneled rooms with two or three benches. The floor used to be hard earth; in later years it was covered with slate and now it is either wood or tile. The heart of the sauna is the heater, which provides the high, dry temperatures for which the Finnish sauna is known.

Cottage saunas, often built near lakes or rivers, provide a perfect setting for the sauna ritual of heat, cold water and fresh air.

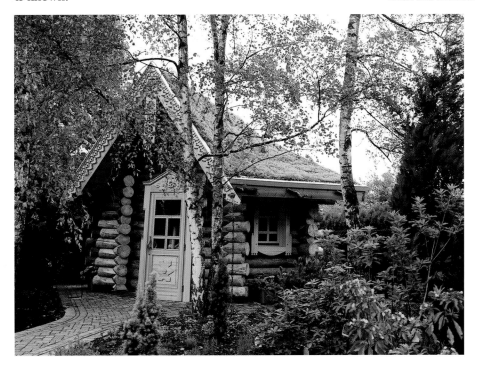

The Tropical Bath, the Dream Sauna and the Bio-Sauna

"To know the Finnish sauna is to know heaven and hell," explained an international traveler after visiting Finland. A lot of people do not like the high, dry sauna temperature because they don't know how to handle it. But often these people make the mistake of sitting on the lowest bench, where they do not enjoy the health benefits outlined earlier. The air is not hot enough at that level to raise the body temperature and sweating is negligible. The humidity at that level is higher as well, and this strains the heart and circulatory system. Instead of feeling refreshed after the sauna people who use it improperly are tired and worn out with no energy. The second bench has a higher temperature and a slightly lower humidity, but sweating is induced. Because it is more comfortable there, time spent in the sauna can be increased.

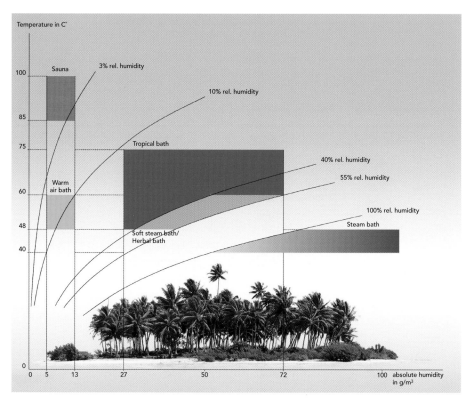

Temperature in C°

Sauna

3% rel. humidity

10% rel. humidity

Tropical bath

40% rel. humidity

55% rel. humidity

100% rel. humidity

Warm air bath

Steam bath

Soft steam bath/ Herbal bath

100   85   75   60   48   40   0

0   5   13   27   50   72   100   absolute humidity in g/m³

Sweating is not as intense as on the third bench, where the temperature reaches around 100°C, but it is still acceptable. To cater to those who prefer a sauna with higher humidity and lower heat, sauna manufacturers developed another type of sauna.

The Bio-Sauna: This type of sauna looks like a wood-paneled Finnish sauna. The temperature is very pleasant, measuring from 40°C (104°F) at the bottom to approximately 75°C (167°F) at the ceiling. Consider this sauna a warm-air bath. The humidity ranges from 40 to 55 percent. The first time I entered a bio-sauna the velvety-soft feeling of the air surprised me. I felt almost immediately relaxed and sleepy. Research released by the Charite Hospital in Berlin indicates that this type of sauna has a gentler effect on the heart and circulation and decreases the blood pressure more moderately. The Bio-Sauna I used featured several lights that changed color capturing my interest and imagination; this type of sauna is also called a "sanarium."

The Dream Sauna: Similar looking to the Bio-Sauna, the Dream Sauna I visited had a wall display mimicking a waterfall and background music with nature sounds. For a Finn these additions to the sauna would probably be annoying. I must say that while I didn't find it annoying, I also prefer my time in the sauna to be quiet. Instead of slipping into that "floating" feeling of relaxation I somehow stayed focused, looking and listening. For others, however, it may be the perfect condition for relaxation.

The Tropical Bath: This is a combination of the Bio-Sauna, the sanarium and the Dream Sauna. While the temperature is close to 50°C (122°F) the humidity is kept at 40 to 60 percent. Sweating is easy because of the high humidity. The use of herbal extracts and aromatic oils add a different dimension to the sauna experience. The tropical bath is considered a soft steam bath. The procedure is the same as in the Finnish sauna: alternating the heat with cold water and cool-down periods, repeated two or three times.

The Steam Bath

One hundred percent humidity at a temperature of 40° to 50°C (104°–122°F) makes sweating easy and immediate, but for some of us breathing is difficult in those conditions.

The steam bath is a room usually completely tiled or consisting of acrylic panels. When stone or tiles are used, the floor and

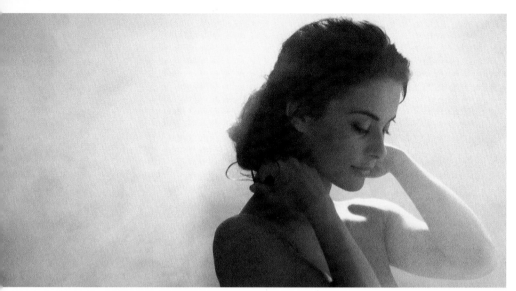

The steam bath is beneficial for relaxation, respiratory disorders and rheumatic pain.

benches are heated to provide the greatest comfort. The steam bath is very popular in Turkey and Russia but has also made a lot of headway in western culture to complement the dry sauna.

The steam bath, with 100 percent humidity, is more than just a room full of mist. It's healthful, too. It's perfect for relaxation and is beneficial for respiratory disorders and rheumatic pain. The humid heat is good for your circulation and cleanses and tones the skin. The heater and evaporator are placed outside the room and with the touch of a button provide a steady stream of mist, to which aromatic oils or fragrances can be added. Temperature control is of utmost importance to avoid being scalded by the steam. This is the major difference between the dry sauna and the steam bath: the sauna's dry 100°C heat and low humidity of 3 to 5 percent do not burn you. Humid heat, experienced in the dry sauna by dousing the hot rocks with water, can be uncomfortable, but in the steam bath, at a humidity of 100 percent, if the heat goes up too high, it will burn you badly.

If you build your own steam bath, an important consideration is the prevention of condensation dripping from the ceiling. Klafs Sauna has developed a special M-shaped roof with a condensation gutter. The ordinary gable roof prevents dripping from the ceiling as well. Often slanted ceilings are built. If you build a steam bath in your house, you must also make sure that the ventilation is perfect, because you don't want the high humidity to escape into your house.

Far-Infrared Saunas

Infrared heat is the radiation from the sun that we enjoy, especially in the early mornings when the air is still cool; you know the feeling. But don't confuse infrared with ultraviolet rays, which are dangerous. Infrared rays are invisible but warm. Now you can enjoy the sun's heat in your sauna with a far-infrared heating unit. All you have to do is plug it in! No special wiring is required.

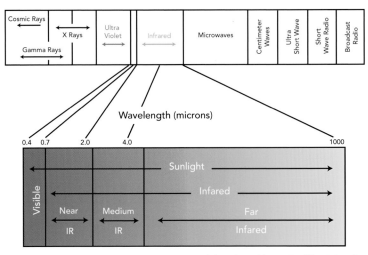

High Tech Health Inc., Boulder, Colorado

The electromagnetic spectrum is divided into three segments by wavelength, which is measured in microns (micrometers). The wavelength of near-infrared light is 0.76 to 1.5 microns, that of middle-infrared is 1.5 to 5.6 microns and far-infrared light has a wavelength of 5.6 to 1000 microns. About 80 percent of the sun's rays are infrared rays. Our body emits infrared heat as well–hold your palms close together but not touching. Can you feel the heat emanating from your hands? Folk healers all over the world use this principle. Heat lamps using the middle-infrared range have been used for many years to heat sore muscles or aching backs and in incubators for premature babies. Far-infrared rays penetrate the body as deeply as 9 centimeters (3.5 inches). Scientists and medical practitioners in Japan and China have been experimenting with far-infrared rays as a heat source in saunas.

Several companies offer simple (no plumbing or special wiring is required), ready-to-assemble far-infrared saunas for home. Health Mate®, Thermal Life® and Soft Heat® are several brands of far-infrared heaters I know of. They work like this: sand in special ceramic tubes is heated by embedded electric coils. A coated metallic grill covers the tube and does not get hot to the touch. Testing by the Swedish National Institute of Radiation Protection revealed no dangerous electromagnetic field around the unit. The temperature range used is between 43° and 55°C (109°–131°F). Sports clubs, clinics and hospitals use the far-infrared sauna because of its simplicity and low operating cost and because very little maintenance is required.

Cabinet Saunas

The horizontal cabinet sauna is a large oblong box (it reminds me of a coffin!) made of durable cedar or similar wood. The top is lifted and closed over you. Your head remains outside the box on a headrest. A towel is wrapped around your neck to keep the heat inside. The heater is located under the center of the box and heats a small basin of water and aromatic herbs. The resulting steam is fed directly into the box. One advantage of this type of sauna is the horizontal position of the body.

This type of sweat bath is used in Ayurvedic healing (the ancient Hindu science of healing and medicine); different herbs

The horizontal cabinet sauna is used in the ancient Hindu science of healing and medicine, known as Ayurvedic healing.

42

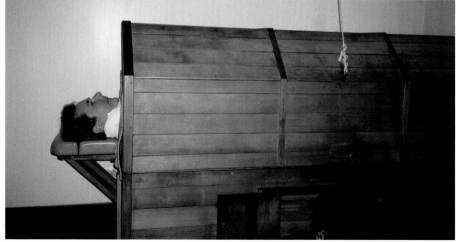

Giselle Roeder

are used to treat different problems. With this type of sauna you also use the cool-down period and sometimes a massage to finish the treatment. For safety's sake, don't use this type of sauna alone; have a knowledgeable and trustworthy person in attendance.

The vertical home cabinet sauna fits into a small corner and was very popular for several years because of its size. It is really a steam bath–you could call it a "sweat box." Sauna aficionados and the International Sauna Association object to it since it is in no way related to the true sauna. The legs are the problem. Because you must remain in a sitting position, with your head outside the box, your leg veins fill up with blood.

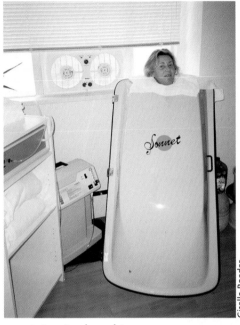

Giselle Roeder

For this type of sauna to be useful, you need to be able to take a really cold shower or a cold-water immersion, do some intensive leg pumping, walk around and then have a rest period lying down with your legs elevated for drainage. You need to do this for the same length of time you spent sitting in the cabinet. There is a danger of falling asleep after this type of sauna (for example, when driving home, etc.) as a result of a shortage of blood and oxygen in your brain because so much of your blood is in your legs. Your blood pressure can drop too low, causing the same problem.

The cabinet sauna is useful for specific health treatments, but not recommended for regular life-long use.

Used with care, this cabinet sauna might have its place for some treatments for a specific period of time, but unlike the traditional sauna it is not recommended for regular life-long use.

A Final Word . . . .

Experiment with sauna types to find the one with which you are most comfortable. Go through the sauna ritual to find what works for you, and make it part of your weekly routine. You will soon reap the health and hygiene benefits enjoyed by Finns and others for centuries!

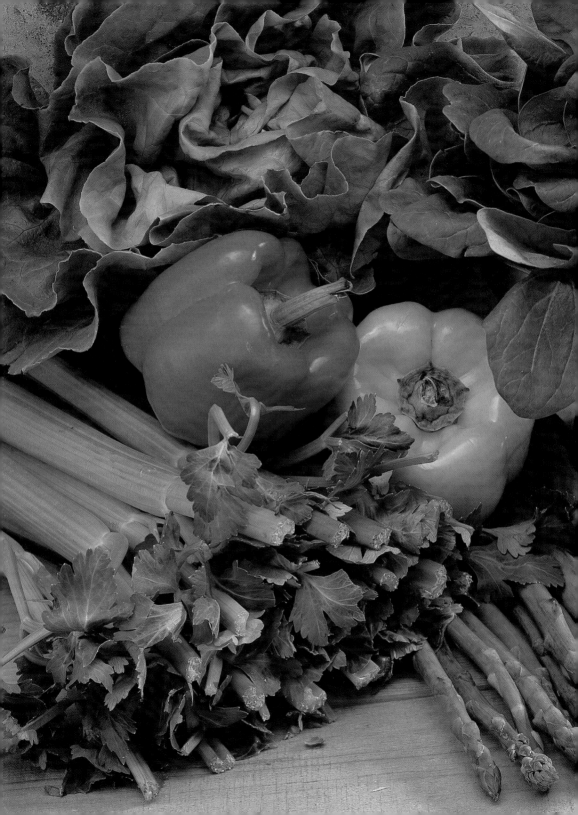

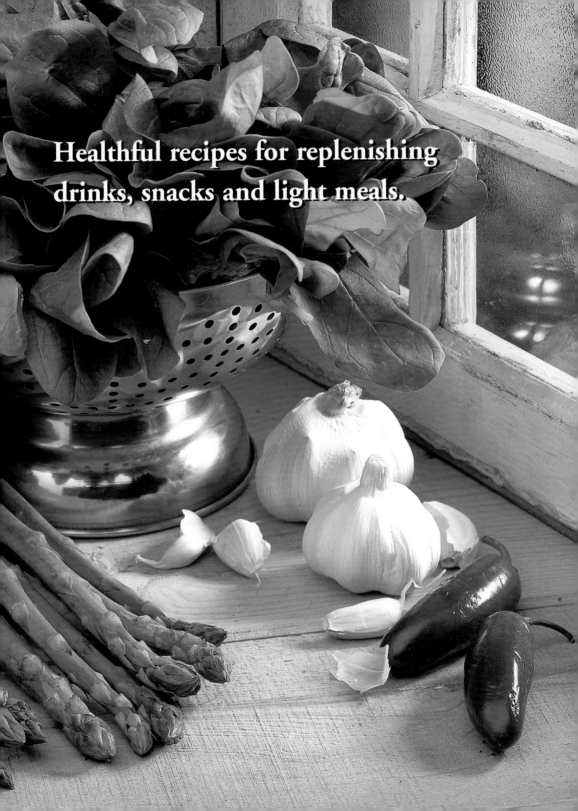

Healthful recipes for replenishing drinks, snacks and light meals.

Fresh Juices

After cooling down and before resting or massage, drinking freshly pressed juices replenishes your fluids and supplies living energy at the same time. Juices are quickly digested, providing a concentration of vitamins, minerals and enzymes.

Drink a selection of these delicious juices at room temperature:
- yellow watermelon - made of 98 percent water
- celery - rich in vitamins and minerals
- cantaloupe - quenches thirst
- red beet - good for the blood and controls blood pressure

Skin Detoxifying Juice

Drinking this cleansing juice keeps your skin glowing with health.

2 raw potatoes	**1 cucumber**
1 green bell pepper	**1 celery stalk or 1 bunch watercress**

Face Cleansing Juice

These refreshing juices clear up pimples and non-infectious blemishes.

4 carrots

1 cucumber

1 whole lemon
(scrape off oily outer skin)

1 raw potato

1 artichoke

1 apple

alternatively

2 apples

1 bunch red grapes

6 apricots (when in season)

For best results prepare about ½ to 1 liter of juice in the morning. Drink equal parts of the juice three times a day. If you are taking the juice for specific ailments it is advisable to take these formulas therapeutically for at least three weeks. You may continue with the therapy as long as you wish, as there are no unpleasant side effects known to any of the formulas. Should you ever find the taste too strong for your palate, dilute the juice with equal parts of water.

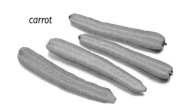

carrot

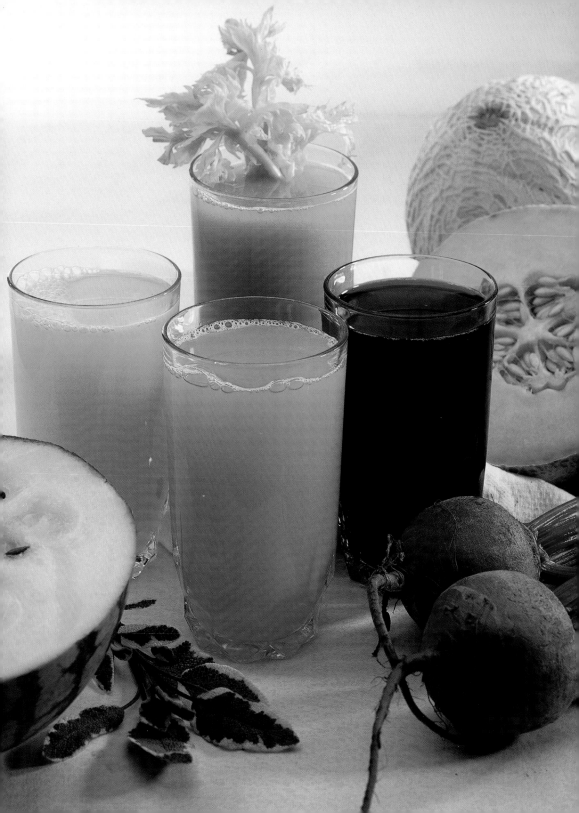

Red Beet and Cabbage Salad

A refreshing light salad is a perfect way to replenish lost fluids, vitamins and minerals. Salads made of raw fruit and vegetables also provide the enzymes important for digestion.

2 cups (500 ml) **red cabbage, shredded**

1 cup (250 ml) **red beets, grated**

1 cup (250 ml) **carrot, shredded** (optional)

1 ½ cups (375 ml) **fresh pineapple, cut in chunks**

2 tbsp extra-virgin olive oil

1 tsp honey

1 tsp fresh rosemary, chopped

In a large bowl, whisk together oil, honey and rosemary. Add cabbage, beet, carrot and pineapple; toss well.

Serves 2

> Substitute carrot with fennel or celery. Both are refreshing and combine well with the other ingredients.

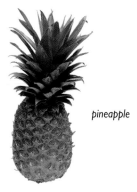

pineapple

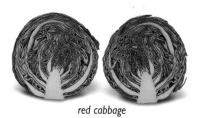

red cabbage

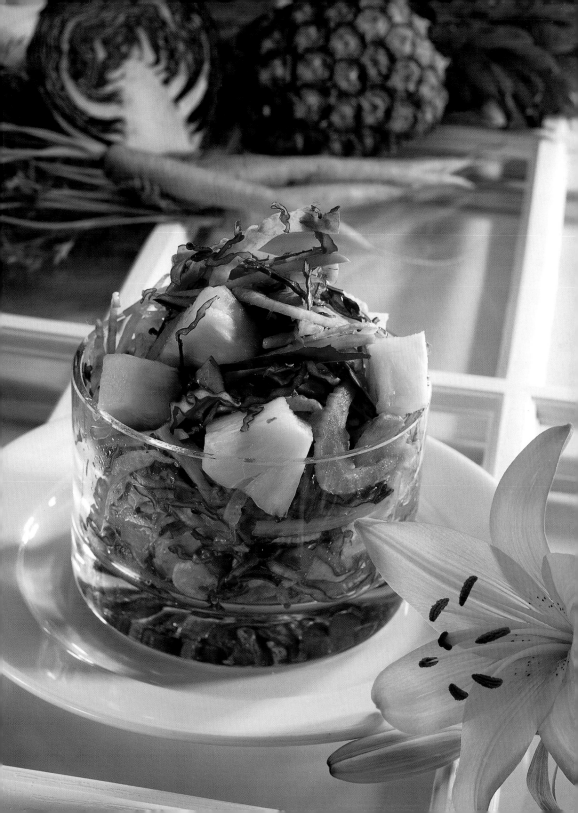

Warm Spinach Salad

Cool your body after coming out of a hot sauna with a refreshing and flavorful combination of spinach, onion and mushroom. The feta replenishes sodium and balsamic reduction provides energy.

2 cups (500 ml) **spinach leaves** (preferably young)

2–3 tbsp feta cheese, crumbled

½ cup (125 ml) **red onion, thinly sliced**

1 ½ cups (375 ml) **mushrooms, stems removed and quartered**

2 tbsp balsamic reduction (see recipe in box)

2 tbsp extra-virgin olive oil

Sea salt, to taste

In a large bowl, whisk together balsamic reduction, oil and salt. Add spinach, feta, onion and mushrooms; toss well. Place salad onto plates, drizzle with extra balsamic reduction, if desired, and serve.

Serves 2

> **Balsamic Reduction**
> In a pan, heat 1 teaspoon of extra-virgin olive oil over medium heat and cook 1 large minced shallot until translucent and it sweats. Add 2 cups (500 ml) of balsamic vinegar, 2 tablespoons of pomegranate syrup (or blackberry jam) and 2 tablespoons of water; reduce by one-third on medium-low heat. Strain. Let cool until thick with a syrup-like consistency.

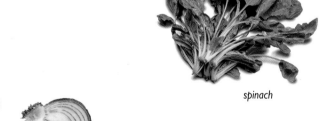

spinach

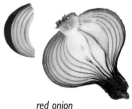

red onion

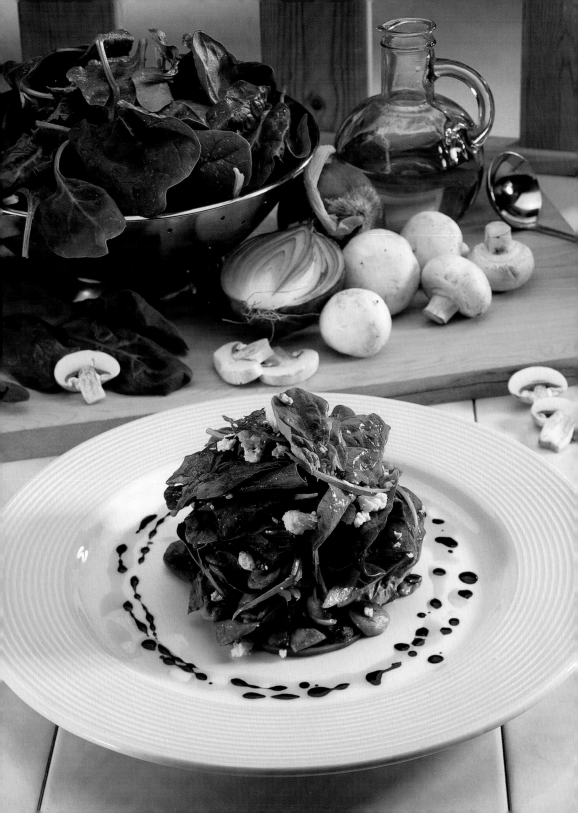

Sushi

Prepared in advance, sushi makes an ideal light lunch or snack after sauna. The seaweed (called nori), captures the taste of the sea, and combined with rice and fresh vegetables, will work to restore the body's balance of vitamins, minerals and water.

4–6 sheets of nori

2 cups (500 ml) **Japanese, jasmine or brown rice, cooked**

1 cup (250 ml) **each red and yellow bell pepper, blanched and julienned**

1 cup (250 ml) **carrot, blanched and julienned**

1 cup (250 ml) **asparagus, blanched and julienned**

1 cup (250 ml) **leek, blanched and julienned**

1 cup (250 ml) **cucumber, julienned**

1 cup (250 ml) **avocado, julienned**

1 cup (250 ml) **radish or other type of sprouts**

Bamboo sushi mat

Tamari, wasabi and pickled ginger

Place each sheet of nori on the bamboo sushi mat, and spread a thin layer of rice on the top, pressing until every corner is covered. On the bottom one-third of the rice, make a dent across then place your choice of julienned vegetables. Start from the bottom and tightly roll the sushi, rolling then pushing back occasionally and pressing each end with the fingertips to keep the vegetables in place. Carefully cut each roll in half, then place the two pieces next to each other lengthwise, and cut in half again. Repeat until there are 8 pieces of equal size. (A wet serrated knife cuts best). Serve with tamari, wasabi and pickled ginger.

Serves 2

> Keep a bowl of water close by and wet your hands when making sushi to prevent the rice from sticking.
>
> Nori is an exceptional source of vitamin A and protein, and high in B, C and D vitamins, calcium, iron, potassium and iodine. It helps break down fats in the body and aids digestion.

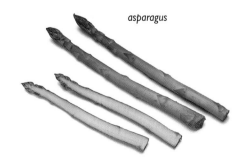

asparagus

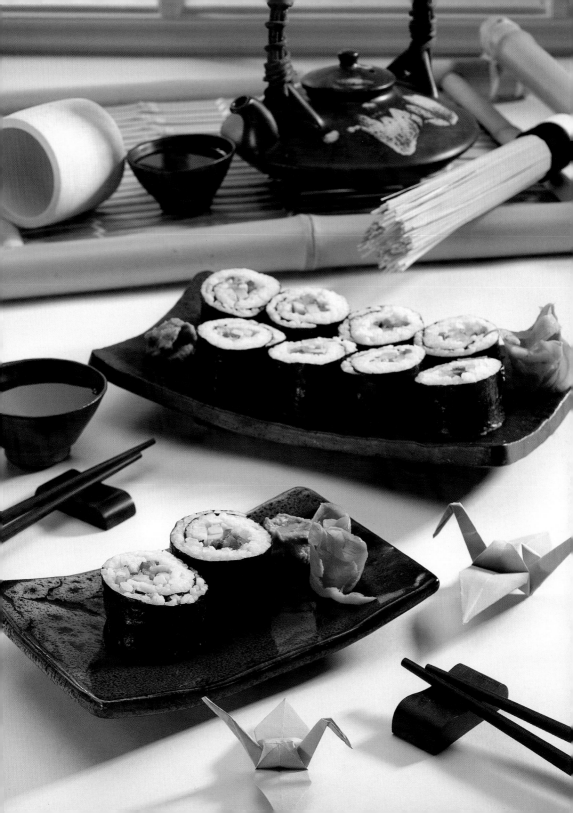

Gazpacho

A traditional soup from Spain, gazpacho was inspired by the hot climate of the Mediterranean. Gazpacho brings down the body temperature on very hot days when the body perspires. It's loaded with taste and nutrition, working to keep you young and happy.

2 lbs (1 kg) **tomato**

1 cup (250 ml) **filtered water**

1 cup (250 ml) **celery, diced**

1 cup (250 ml) **red onion, diced**

1 cup (250 ml) **fennel, diced**

1 cup (250 ml) **each red, yellow and green bell pepper, diced**

¼ cup (60 ml) **extra-virgin olive oil**

3 tbsp fresh lemon juice

1 tsp fresh tarragon, chopped

Pinch cracked chili

Herbamare, to taste

1 tbsp capers (optional)

Cut a small cross shape on the bottom the each tomato. Place tomatoes in a pot of boiling water for 30 seconds then remove them and peel. Remove seeds. Place tomatoes in a blender and purée. Add filtered water and blend again.

In a large bowl, combine tomato purée and remaining ingredients. Season with Herbamare and add capers, if desired. Refrigerate for 1 to 2 hours before serving, in order for the flavors to incorporate.

Serves 2

> Hot peppers and chili are used widely in the Mediterranean—when eaten, body temperature rises and then the breeze cools the body down.

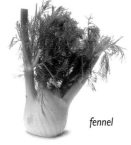

fennel

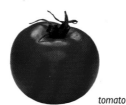

tomato

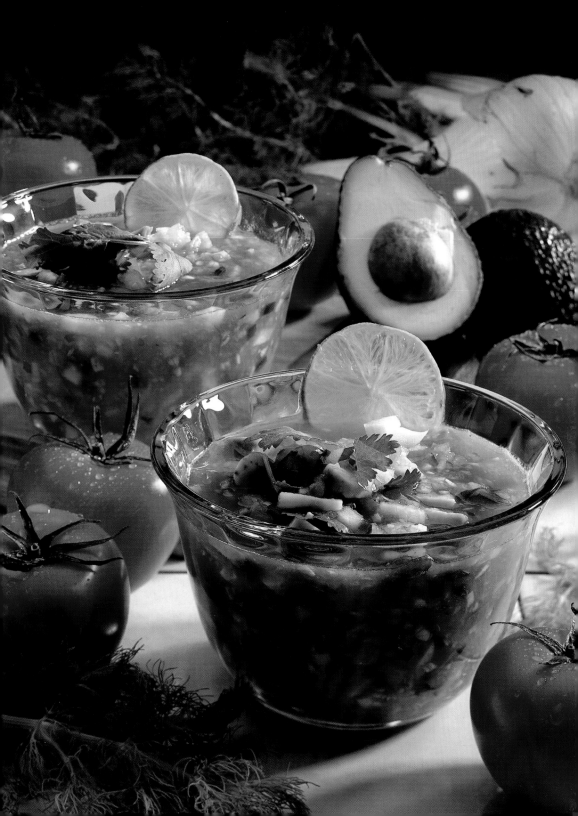

Mushroom-Leek Soup

The mushrooms absorb and enhance the flavors of leek and onion to make a delectable soup that will energize and replenish your mineral and water supply after sauna.

1 lb (500 g) **mushrooms**

2 cups (500 ml) **leeks, sliced**

1 cup (250 ml) **white onion, diced**

2 cloves garlic, minced

2 tbsp + 2 tbsp extra-virgin olive oil

2 cups (500 ml) **vegetable stock**

2 cups (500 ml) **light cream** (half and half)

2 tbsp béchamel sauce

1 tbsp fresh dill, chopped

In a large pot, heat 2 tablespoons of oil over medium heat and briefly sauté mushroom, 1 cup (250 ml) of leek, onion and garlic. Add vegetable stock, salt and pepper; cover and cook for 15 minutes. Strain mushrooms, carefully reserving the liquid, and blend the mushrooms in a food processor until smooth. Return mushrooms and liquid to the pot then add cream and heat on low for 5 minutes or heated through.

In the meantime, sauté remaining leek in oil until soft. Stir in béchamel and dill and serve garnished with leek.

Serves 2

> **Béchamel Sauce**
> Here's a healthy way of preparing a tasty bechamel sauce. Béchamel binds and thickens the soup. You can also use 2 potatoes, cooked and mashed.
> In a pan, dry roast 2 tablespoons each of unbleached and whole wheat flour for 2 minutes over medium heat. The flour should be light yellow, not brown. Reduce heat to low then add 2 tablespoons of butter and stir, smoothing out any clumps. Slowly add 1 cup (250 ml) of milk then 1 cup (250 ml) of water, stirring. Increase heat, bring to a boil then immediately remove from heat.

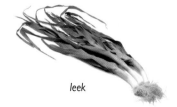

leek

white onion

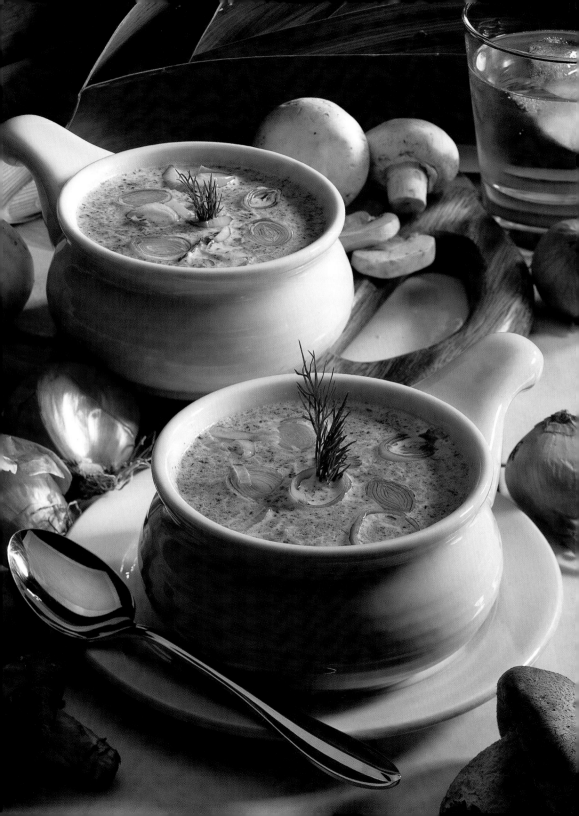

Rice-Vegetable Confetti
with Pineapple

Tangy and fragrant pineapple, along with ginger, starts your digestive juices in a fresh salad that's filling, easy to digest and rich in vitamins, minerals, carbohydrates and fiber.

2 cups (500 ml) **rice, such as long grain or wild, cooked**

⅔ cup (165 ml) **fresh pineapple, diced**

¼ cup (60 ml) **each red and yellow bell pepper, diced**

¼ cup (60 ml) **broccoli florets**

¼ cup (60 ml) **carrot, diced**

¼ cup (60 ml) **celery, diced**

¼ cup (60 ml) **red onion, diced**

¼ cup (60 ml) **extra-virgin olive oil**

1 tbsp fresh lemon juice

1 tbsp orange rind, finely sliced

1 tbsp fresh dill, chopped

2 cloves garlic, minced

1 tsp fresh ginger, minced

Pineapple shells, for garnish

In a large bowl, whisk together oil, lemon juice, orange rind, dill, garlic, ginger and salt. Add rice, pineapple, bell peppers, broccoli, carrot, celery and onion; mix well. Stuff mixture into pineapple shells and serve.

Serves 2

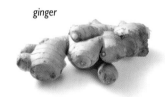

ginger

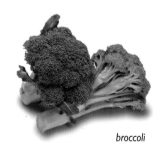

broccoli

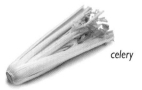

celery

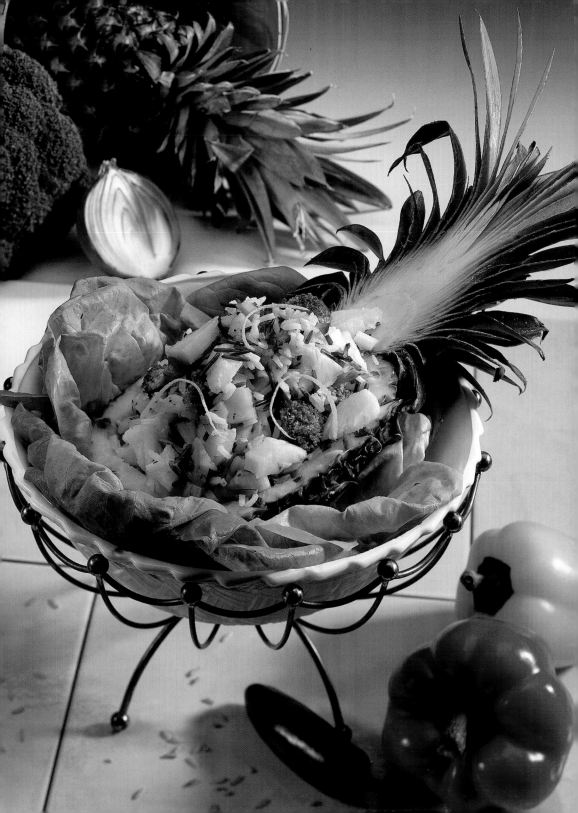

Snapper with Avocado Salsa

This one dish you can count on to replenish your store of potassium after a sauna session. You will gain potassium from the sweet potato, iron from spinach and many other nutrients from the fresh tangy salsa. Fish is not only a great source of protein, it also contains essential fatty acids, sodium and other minerals.

2 red snapper filets (⅔ lbs or 310 g in total), **cut in half**

¼ cup (60 ml) **whole grain bread crumbs**

1 tbsp flax seeds (optional)

1 egg, beaten

2 tbsp whole wheat flour

1 bunch baby spinach

¼ cup (60 ml) **extra-virgin olive oil**

2 cloves garlic, minced

1 small shallot, diced

2 cups (500 ml) **sweet potato, cubed**

Fresh parsley or chives, chopped, for garnish

Salsa:

¼ cup (60 ml) **avocado, diced small**

¼ cup (60 ml) **red onion, diced small**

¼ cup (60 ml) **ripe tomatoes, diced small**

¼ cup (60 ml) **pitted black olives, diced small**

3 tbsp extra-virgin olive oil or flax oil

1 tbsp fresh lemon juice

Preheat the oven at 375°F (190°C).

Place flour on a plate. In a bowl, beat egg well. On another plate, mix together bread crumb and flax seeds.

Dip filets in the flour, then in the egg wash and last in the bread crumbs. In an ovenproof pan, heat 2 tablespoons of oil over medium heat and brown each side for 1 minute. Bake in the oven for 5 minutes or until done.

In the meantime, sauté spinach, garlic and shallot in 1 tablespoon of oil until just wilted. Season with salt and pepper. Blanch sweet potato in a pot of boiling salted water for 5 to 7 minutes. Drain and rinse with cold water.

To prepare the salsa, combine avocado, onion, tomato and olives in a bowl. Add oil and lemon juice; toss well.

Place sweet potato onto plates and drizzle with 1 tablespoon of olive oil. Arrange spinach and snapper on top. Serve with a dollop of salsa and fresh parsley.

Serves 2

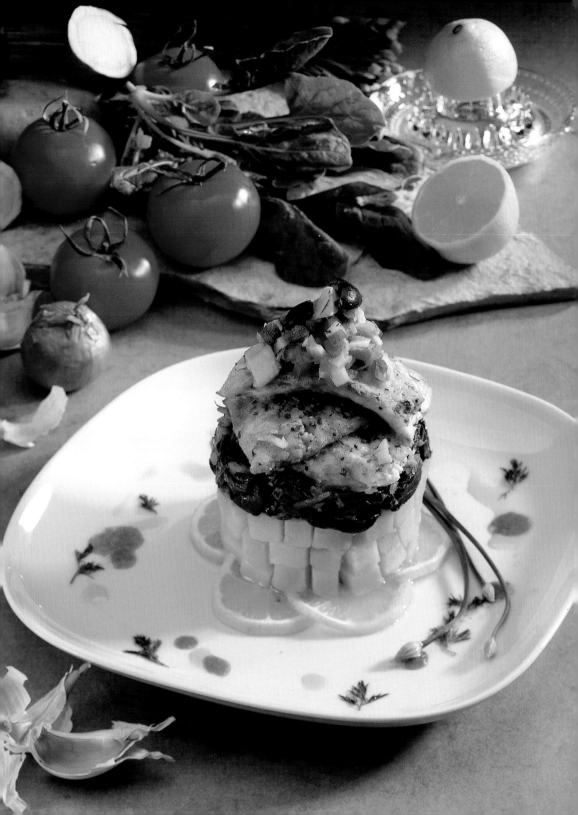

Whole Wheat Pita-Pizza

Eat a light meal after a sauna–do not overeat. Cayenne is one of the best plant sources of vitamin C and is very important for cleansing as it has sweat-inducing properties.

2 whole wheat pita breads

2 to 3 tbsp extra-virgin olive oil

Generous dash cayenne pepper

2 cups (500 ml) **mixed julienned vegetables such as red, yellow, green bell peppers, red onion, carrot, avocado, fennel, daikon**

1 clove garlic, sliced

Broccoli florets

10–12 slices camembert cheese

1 small or ½ large banana, sliced

1 small tomato, sliced

Leaves of romaine lettuce, for garnish

Preheat oven to 350°F (180°C).

In a bowl, combine oil and cayenne. Add mixed vegetables and garlic; toss well. Blanch broccoli in a pot of boiling salted water for 1 minute to bring out the bright color.

Place julienned vegetables onto pita then arrange broccoli in the middle and cheese slices around. Bake for 10 minutes or until cheese melts. Remove from oven, arrange banana slices around, garnish with tomato and serve on a bed of lettuce.

Serves 2

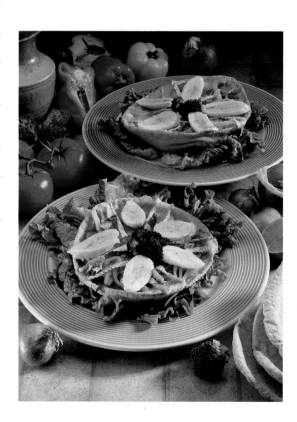

sources

Erlebnisbad 'aquaria'
Alpenstrasse 5
87534 Oberstaufen/
Germany
Tel:+49-8386-931-30
Fax: 08386-9313-40
www.aquaria.de
Email: Info@aquaria.de

Vital Zentrum
Felbermayer
A-6793 Gaschurn im
Alpenpark Montafon
Austria
Tel: +43-5558-8617-0
Fax: –8617-41
www.vital-zentrum.at
Email:
info@vital-zentrum.at

Klafs Saunabau
G.m.b.H. & Co.
Dipl.Ing. Stefan Schoell-
hammer
Erich-Klafs-Strasse 1 – 3
74523 Schwaebisch
Hall/Germany
Tel: +49-791-5010
Fax: +49-791-5012-48
www.klafs.de
Email:
susanne.radtke@klafs.de

The O3 Zone
Health Spa
Peter Morrow,
17267 – 24th Avenue
White Rock BC. V4P 2V2
Tel: 604-535-4606

West Coast College of
Massage Therapy
Harbour Center 6th Floor
Spencer Building
555 West Hastings Street,
Vancouver BC. V6B 4N6
Tel: 604-685-5801
www.icchc.edu/

Natural Solutions,
Randy Gomm, B.Sc.
Tel: 604-292-8252
Fax: 604-291-8286
www.infraredsauna.net
Email:
randy@infraredsauna.net

High Tech Health, Inc.
Thermal Life Far Infrared
Sauna Therapy,
2695 Linden Drive,
Boulder, CO
80304-0450 USA
Tel: 303-413-8500
Fax: 303-449-9640
Toll-Free: 1-800-794-5355
www.hightechhealth.com

for healthy oils:

Flora
7400 Fraser Park Drive
Burnaby BC V5J 5B9
(604) 436–6000
1-800–663–0617
(Western Canada)
1-800–387–7541
(Eastern Canada)

Gold Top Organics
16831-110 Ave.
Edmonton, Alberta
Tel/Fax: 780-483-1504
Toll Free: 1-877-891-4019

Omega Nutrition of
Canada, Inc.
1924 Franklin Street
Vancouver BC V5L 1R2
Tel: 604-253-4677
Toll Free: 1-800–661–3529
www.omegaflo.com

Omega–Life, Inc.
15355 Woodridge Road
Brookfield, WI 53005
Tel: (414) 786–2070
Toll Free: 1–800–328–3529
(1–800–EAT–FLAX)

Remedies and supplements mentioned in this book are
available at quality health food stores and nutrition centers.

First published in 2001 by
alive **books**
7436 Fraser Park Drive
Burnaby BC V5J 5B9
(604) 435–1919
1-800–661–0303

© 2001 by *alive* books

613.41
ROE
H
1/6/11

Book Design:
    Liza Novecoski
Artwork:
    Terence Yeung
    Raymond Cheung
Food Styling/Recipe Development:
    Fred Edrissi
Photography:
    KLAFS (except when credited otherwise)
Recipe Photography:
    Edmond Fong
Photo Editing:
    Sabine Edrissi-Bredenbrock
Editing:
    Sandra Tonn
    Donna Dawson

Canadian Cataloguing in
Publication Data

Giselle Roeder
    Sauna: The Hottest Way to
    Good Health

(*alive* Natural Health Guides, 32
ISSN 1490-6503)
ISBN 1-55312-034-5

Printed in Canada

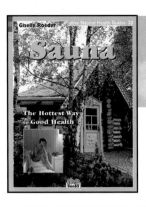

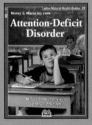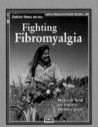
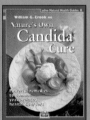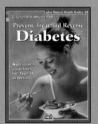
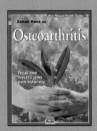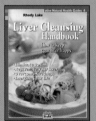
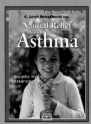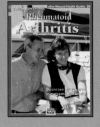
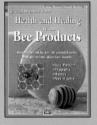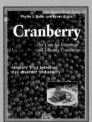
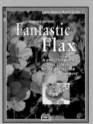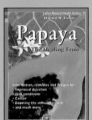
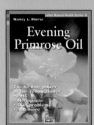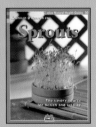
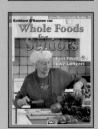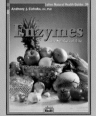